Canetha Amour-Porter's

For The Love
of Family

How I healed my Family's Skin
from my Kitchen!

For The Love Of Family

<u>FOREWORD</u>

It was 2010, a beautiful weekend in Michigan where I had the distinct pleasure of meeting Canetha Amour-Porter. We both held high-ranking positions in a health and wellness company. Even though we were only acquaintances at that time, she amplified a presence that showed compassion that always ignited the room. When Canetha would speak, her presentation was flawless. Cleary, she was definitely a woman about her business, bold and beautiful.

One day I received an email, and it said you might not remember me, but we were in the same company a few years ago. Little to her surprise, I knew exactly who she was. What she did not know,

For The Love Of Family

I admired her business, boldness, and beauty from afar. There is a saying the old folks would say, "You never know who is watching you." She had been watching me this time, and I never knew. Therefore, that statement is authentic and often wondered where Canetha went after all those years.

During our many conversations, I learned we both went to establish our own companies. Canetha developed a company Amour Your Body LLC, not to my surprise, where she was healing her family with love from her kitchen. She has an excellent product that helps people with skin disorders. This product has been presented to HSN and offered in many store outlets. Canetha shared her product with me, and it works wonders on dry skin. My skin is dry due to medications, and it is soothing to the skin and relieves dryness. As Canetha's business continues to help families with skin disorders from her kitchen, I am sure this will be a million-dollar baby soon.

It is with great honor to reconnect with Canetha Amour-Porter, not as an acquaintance, but a true testament to being a business colleague and a friend. Congratulations on your book and many more to come.

Dr. Missy Johnson

Fearless Women Rock LLC

For The Love Of Family

Testimonials

Here are just a few of our testimonials:

I'm super addicted to this body butter. I have lavender, and the lemon and eucalyptus. As a baker, I wash my hands a lot. This helps keep my hands from cracking, and I don't have to keep reapplying it constantly. My husband has recently discovered it and is using it now too every day. Amazing stuff!

~Erika Helwig

Love Love Love this amazing product!! I am a licensed massage therapist, and I now use this product on many of my clients with sensitive skin. They are amazed at how smooth it feels; it also nourishes the skin issues they may have when they come in for their massage!! Many amazing fragrances to choose from as well, beautiful product!!

~Michelle Koester

BodyMax Massage

For The Love Of Family

Yesterday I had a massage, the masseuse placed oil on my back and start massaging and it felt cool but yet had a warm sensation along with the coolness made the massage more amazing. I asked about the oil and her response, "Do you like it, it's your daughters!" Thanks Canetha for making my massage more amazing!

~Katherine J (Mom)

I took the Amour Your Body cream to Mexico and used it on my skin after being in the sun!! I didn't peel, and it also relieved the sunburn on my shoulders!! The burn just faded in one day as a tan!! Love this product!!

~Therese Bosek Ercolani

I have combination skin, meaning some parts of my face get really dry at times. When I started using this, it helps moisturize those parts of my face, and it has improved my skin a lot!
Also, a little goes a long way. I have been using it for 3 months now, and I still have half a jar left.

For The Love Of Family

~Alexandria Amour

"I just love the Amour Your Body Butter. My husband and I were so excited to get our full size "tub" today. Can't wait to use it, especially since we had run out of our sample size. We are very particular about what we put on and in our body, and as someone who makes her own body butter, I can tell you Amour's is among the best—deliciously luxurious. It's so silky and gives excellent moisturizing coverage all day long without being oily. Win-win! We got the Lemongrass version and it smells heavenly, but not too fragrant as to give us a headache. We absolutely love it. Treat yourself to some of this buttery gold!"

~ The McDonalds, Woodbridge, VA

I AM LOVING THE BODY CREAM! The smell is fantastic and a little goes a long way. It melts beautifully into your skin and easily lasts all day. My skin is pretty resilient, but my daughter gets rashes, bites, and redness all the time. I used the cream on a rash that she got out of nowhere and it healed in no time! Miracle Cream! You have to try it!

For The Love Of Family

~Chelsea Elisa

My skin is so in LOVE!!…now if I can get my co-workers out of my jar, lol. It's in the Name! Your skin will love it!

~Chantal Whitman

I need to replenish my supply!…This butter is THE TRUTH! It passed the ultimate test… my 4-year-old's knees were the same color when he came home from school today, as they were when he left the house this morning. #winning #grayisnotcute

~Gloria Raines

I absolutely love the silky smoothness of Amour Body Butter! It helps my psoriasis from itching and flaking, and leaves my skin well moisturized! Thank you, Amour Your Body!

~Sarah

For The Love Of Family

So I have been using this product on specific areas of my body. With Fall season here, and Winter approaching, my eczema flares up this time of the year. I stopped using steroid medicines a long time ago, and it is difficult to find creams that truly work. What I love about this product is that it is clearing up spots that I have had for a long time. It doesn't burn when I apply it to the area. It is not greasy, smells wonderful! Plus, Organic! This is a Win all the way around. I am going to try this also as a deep conditioner in my hair! Can't wait to see those results as well! Love this product!

~Emily

This body butter is absolutely amazing! I have acne on my back and have suffered through scratching fits for years. I didn't know that it was possible for me to have total relief until now! I am completely hooked. Let me encourage you, TRY IT! You will NOT regret it!

~Ian

For The Love Of Family

I just tried Amour Your Body Butter for the first time... all I can say is WOW! I have not found a product that is so light but had continuous moisture. I love everything about it, it made my skin hydrated, silky smooth, loved the texture, the scent, and that it was natural and oh so good for your skin! I need to order this by the vat full. I do not want to be without this wonderful product. You can tell this body butter was handcrafted with LOVE! You have a forever customer!

~Rita

The "Amour Your Body" Experience

This product is really WONDERFUL. I recently purchased the body butter in both the Original and Clean scents. The other benefit was that the proprietor offered to create a custom scent of my liking!

That was an added and rare incentive! What I found fascinating was that I could lather it on after a morning bath and how it continued to cling to my skin throughout the entire day. My skin remained soft and smooth by bedtime, as well!

For The Love Of Family

Also, using the butter as a hair mask when conditioning gave my hair volume and left it so soft! That's awesome, considering that many products have an adverse or hardening effects on African-American hair. So whether it's for your epidermis or mane, you'll love Amour Your Body! It's great to use something that is chemical-free and simply natural!

~Della

Table of Contents	Page

Disclaimer

This book or eBook contains information that is intended to help the readers be better-informed about consumers of healthcare products. It is presented as general advice on health care products. Always consult your doctor for your individual needs.

Limit of Liability/Disclaimer of Warranty: Resultsof our products may vary from person to person with the use of Amour Your Body, LLC products. This book is not intended as a substitute for the medical advice of physicians, Nor dores it suggest that the information written here in or the use of Amour Your Body, LLC products, will result in the healing of skin disorders. the reader should regularly consult a physician on matters relating to his/her health and particularly with respect to any symptoms that may require diagnosis or medical attention.

For The Love Of Family

<u>Introduction</u>

I'm a mom and wife who just wants the best for my family. That is why, after many years of doctor/dermatologist appointments and prescription medicine for our many skin sensitivities and disorders, I decided to do something different.

I decided to learn about natural ingredients and essential oils and how they can protect and heal our skin, and by goll, I did just that! After years of experimentation, I found the right formula. I developed a cream that is not only sensitive enough to use on our problem skin, but it's also a great moisturizer for normal skin.

For The Love Of Family

Amour Your Body Cream, was created out of love, in my own kitchen. Now I'm sharing my creation of love with you and your family.

Amour Your Body body cream, is made with all natural oils. This is why we say, "Amour Your Body with a gift of nature." You're going to love Amour Your Body cream!

Amour Your Body body Cream has helped my family and many others with:

- Eczema,
- Dermatitis
- Psoriasis
- Face Protector before Makeup for Sensitive Skin
- Dry Skin
- Soften Skin and Feet

For The Love Of Family

- Hair and Scalp Dryness

- UV Protectant

- Skin Elasticity

- Insect Repellant

- A great hair conditioner and much more!

You have read testimony after testimony from people who uses our products, now here's how it started...

<u>The Beginning</u>

Growing up, I never thought I had a skin disorder. I knew that I had more than the average amount of dandruff, but never thought that my excessive amounts of dandruff were a symptom of a skin disorder. My parents and I didn't think too much about it. I would have my dandruff scratched and hair washed more than usual as an African American girl. As I got older, I started using chemicals in my hair. Soon, I started developing raw patches on my face, in my scalp, and on my ears. I knew this wasn't good and sought help.

I went to a dermatologist to find out what was going on with my skin. I was told that it was from the chemicals I was using and that my skin would go back to normal when I stopped using them. I was prescribed topical steroids and was sent on my way.

I stopped using the harmful chemicals in my hair, and my skin cleared up. That is until the next outbreak. See, at that time, I still didn't know that I have a skin disorder and that stress, drastic weather changes, and some foods cause my skin to constantly break out. I live in Michigan, and the weather is forever changing. It wasn't until I had been visiting a dermatologist for years, using all types of medicines that didn't really work that I decided to figure out a better way for heal my skin.

Don't get me wrong, I have a great respect for doctors and their profession. I just feel that it's our duty to understand and learn our own bodies. No one will ever know your body as well as you will. We have to start listening to what our body is telling us.

When I took the time to start noticing when my breakouts occurred and what was going on with my body, I was able to tell the next doctor what to look for. Finally, I was diagnosed correctly. See, it's not just the doctor's job to diagnose you, you have to take part in your own health and well-being.

Now that I knew what was going on with my body, I could choose what methods I would use to heal my skin. If I knew my breakout was caused by drastic weather change and I knew that the weather would stabilize soon, I could choose to just keep it moisturized and that my skin would regulate itself in the next few days. Being able to take control of my own skin health is something that I cherish to this day.

The Curve Ball

Life was good. I knew that I could never get rid of my skin disorder, but I could maintain it and have fewer severe outbreaks. My 2 older children had perfect skin. No issues. But shortly after my youngest daughter was born, I started seeing rashes on her body and inflammation on her skin.

Oh no! What to do? I never experienced this. My skin disorder started on my scalp and went down to my face and ears, but it never spread any further. I knew how to take care of the skin disorder I have, but this was something different.

I was devastated, seeing my baby girl go through this. I couldn't stop the pain and uncomfortableness she was experiencing. We took her to the doctor, and they said that she had Eczema. That's when my husband said that he also had eczema as a child. He thought he had grew out of it but he has flare-ups very rarley. We searched for different remedies because we didn't want to give our daughter harmful medicines.

Around the same time the following year, our infant son started experiencing signs of eczema. While his symptoms were not as severe as his sisters, he still had some pain and uncomfortableness. So here, I am with 4 children and 2 of them with Eczema.

<u>The Visits</u>

This was our season of doctor and dermatologist appointments. Four young children with regular checkups and vaccination appointments can keep any mother extremely busy. Now, add in dermatologist appointments, it was a crazy-busy time in our life.

One of the things I hated in this period in our lives was that I was buying 3 to 4 different creams for the family and they were all expensive. My youngest two children had two different types of severities, so they used two different creams.

I has diagnosed with Dermatitis.this made it necessary that I used a different type of moisturizer than the rest of my family. A few years later, my youngest daughter started having a rash on her leg and loss of pigmentation on her fingers. Oh no, I thought to myself. What could this be? So I scheduled a dermatologist appointment. At the appointment, we discovered that she has Psoriasis and Vitiligo along with Dermatitis. I was devastated. I couldn't imagine how she felt being so your with skin disorders.

No mother wants her child to have to deal with this, and at such a young age. While we were at the appointment, the doctor explained that there was a medicine that could clear up her skin. There were just a few side effects, which were depression and thoughts of suicide. In that moment, being concerned about my child, his words didn't register.

Because of my state of mind, I didn't really think about what was just said, and I took the prescription intending to get it filled. On the ride home, I said to myself, "What did that doctor just say to me about the side effects of this medicine he just prescribed?" I remember thinking to myself, saying there is no way that I will ever give her this medicine.

My Aha Moment

At this moment in my life, I felt like I had lost control and I needed to gain it back for my family's health. I started looking at the products at the health food stores. They had products that were all natural, but we either didn't like the smell or the texture of the creams. They were expensive, and I had to buy different types of creams for our four different skin disorders and that didn't even include the moisturizer needed for the other half of my family.

After being excited about finding these products, I quickly became frustrated when they didn't solve all of our problems. Plus, buying all of these different products was costly, throwing our budget out of whack. I knew I had to try to do something to help my family that wouldn't leave us broke and having nothing to fully help our skin disorders. I decided to create something my whole family could use. I had some knowledge of what natural products could work due to the research I did when I was looking for products years ago, which I used to help my skin.

I started with 100% pure Shea Butter. I knew that this would protect our skin. I researched more about how our bodies work and what our skin needed to become healthier. Shea Butter has so many wonderful properties, and it is naturally rich in vitamins A, E, and F. Shea Butter is a UV protectant (SPF ~6) and infuses your skin with essential fatty acids and the nutrients necessary for collagen production. From there, I personally chose only the best ingredients to give my family nothing but the very best.

Now, I'm not saying that I healed us from the actual skin disorder itself. I can't do that. What I am saying is that using my Amour Your Body, body cream healed our skin when It was broken, blistered, and covered with rashes. I can say that the daily use of our products has caused outbreaks to occur less often and with less severity.

That's a win-win for us and it will be for you! You don't have to live life in pain or irritation. You don't have to worry about having broken skin from scratching affected areas with the daily use of our products. You also don't have to worry about using oils and creams made from chemicals that may be harmful to your skin.

Amour Your Body, body cream was created with ingredients that are all-natural ingredients my own family uses on a daily basis.

Amour Your Body, body cream is made in my kitchen, For The Love Of My Family.

Conclusion

There are so many Americans suffering from Eczema, Psoriasis, and Dermatitis, looking for a way to ease the pain and soothe their skin without harmful prescription medicines. Our company gives them an all-natural option that is safe enough for babies and strong enough to use on old, scarred, and swelled skin.

Our company was started because 5 out of 7 people in my household have some type of skin disorder where steroids and other medicine didn't work, or the side effects were harmful. For years, I studied the body and created a formula that healed our skin and now helps others.

We have many wonderful testimonies of how our products have soothed and healed the skin of all kinds of people and our products have changed their lives. Because I know what my cream has done for me and my family, I want to help more people know that there's an amazing product that is waiting to help them stop suffering. Don't Wait! Amour Your Body and Start Your Healing Today!

www.AmourYourBody.com

<u>Note From My Mother</u>

It goes without saying that I'm proud of Canetha, but what needs to be said is that Canetha has an unstoppable spirit for those who have not seen her in action. To have an unstoppable spirit, married, with a heart to help people, it equals to an awesome and outstanding person! So when it came to her children having skin disorders, I knew she would be vigilant with love as the undertone to find an answer for her children's discomfort. When she couldn't find the answer, she developed it, and that is what makes my daughter so awesome!

Love Mom

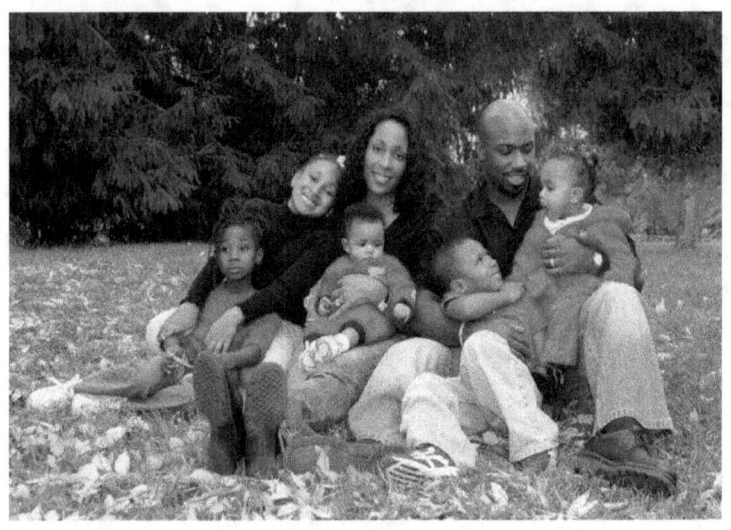

This is a picture of Canetha, Toc and children in the early years.